I0409688

ALCOHOL

A Women's Health Issue

Table of Contents

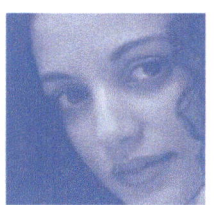 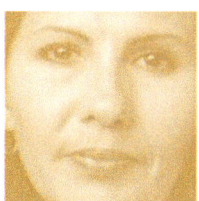 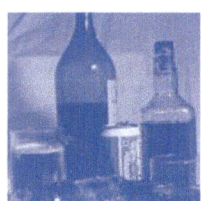 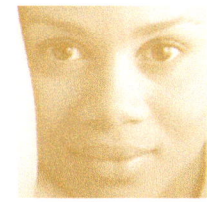 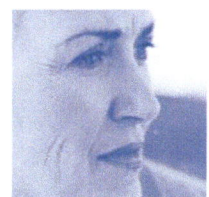

WOMEN AND DRINKING

Exercise, diet, hormones, and stress: keeping up with all the health issues facing women is a challenge.

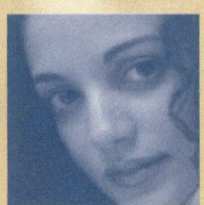

Alcohol presents yet another health challenge for women. Even in small amounts, alcohol affects women differently than men. In some ways, heavy drinking is much more risky for women than it is for men.

With any health issue, accurate information is key. There are times and ways to drink that are safer than others. Every woman is different. No amount of drinking is 100 percent safe, 100 percent of the time, for every woman. With this in mind, it's important to know how alcohol can affect a woman's health and safety.

How Much Is Too Much?

Sixty percent of U.S. women have at least one drink a year. Among women who drink, 13 percent have more than seven drinks per week.

For women, this level of drinking is above the recommended limits published in the *Dietary Guidelines for Americans,* which are issued jointly by the U.S. Department of Agriculture and the U.S. Department of Health and Human Services. (The *Dietary Guidelines* can be viewed online at www.nutrition.gov.)

The *Dietary Guidelines* define moderate drinking as no more than one drink a day for women and no more than two drinks a day for men.

The *Dietary Guidelines* point out that drinking more than one drink per day for women can increase the risk for motor vehicle crashes, other

> **What is a drink? A standard drink is:**
>
> One 12-ounce bottle of beer or wine cooler
>
> One 5-ounce glass of wine
>
> 1.5 ounces of 80-proof distilled spirits
>
> Keep in mind that the alcohol content of different types of beer, wine, and distilled spirits can vary quite substantially.

injuries, high blood pressure, stroke, violence, suicide, and certain types of cancer.

Some people should not drink at all, including:

- Anyone under age 21
- People of any age who are unable to restrict their drinking to moderate levels
- Women who may become pregnant or who are pregnant
- People who plan to drive, operate machinery, or take part in other activities that require attention, skill, or coordination
- People taking prescription or over-the-counter medications that can interact with alcohol.

Why are lower levels of drinking recommended for women than for men? Because women are at greater risk than men for developing alcohol-related problems. Alcohol passes through the digestive tract and is dispersed in the water in the body. The more water available, the more diluted the alcohol. As a rule, men weigh more than women, and, pound for pound, women have less water in their bodies than men. Therefore, a woman's brain and other organs are exposed to more alcohol and to more of the toxic byproducts that result when the body breaks down and eliminates alcohol.

Moderate Drinking: Benefits and Risks

Moderate drinking can have short- and long-term health effects, both positive and negative:

- **Benefits**

  Heart disease: Once thought of as a threat mainly to men, heart disease also is the leading killer of women in the United States. Drinking moderately may lower the risk for coronary heart disease, mainly among women over age 55. However, there are other factors that reduce the risk of heart disease, including a healthy diet, exercise, not smoking, and keeping a healthy weight. Moderate drinking provides little, if any, net health benefit for younger people. (Heavy drinking can actually damage the heart.)

- **Risks**

  Drinking and driving: It doesn't take much alcohol to impair a person's ability to drive. The chances of being killed in a single-vehicle crash are increased at a blood alcohol level that a 140-lb. woman would reach after having one drink on an empty stomach.

  Medication interactions: Alcohol can interact with a wide variety of medicines, both prescription and over-the-counter. Alcohol can reduce the effectiveness of some medications, and it can combine with other medications to cause or increase side effects. Alcohol can interact with medicines used to treat conditions as varied as heart and blood vessel disease, digestive problems, and diabetes. In particular, alcohol can increase the sedative effects of any medication that causes drowsiness, including cough and cold medicines and drugs for anxiety and depression. **When taking any medication, read package labels and warnings carefully.**

Breast cancer: Research suggests that as little as one drink per day can slightly raise the risk of breast cancer in some women, especially those who are postmenopausal or have a family history of breast cancer. It is not possible, however, to predict how alcohol will affect the risk for breast cancer in any one woman.

Fetal Alcohol Syndrome: Drinking by a pregnant woman can harm her unborn baby, and may result in a set of birth defects called fetal alcohol syndrome (FAS).

Fetal Alcohol Syndrome

Fetal alcohol syndrome (FAS) is the most common known preventable cause of mental impairment. Babies with FAS have distinctive changes in their facial features and they may be born small. The brain damage that occurs with FAS can result in lifelong problems with learning, memory, attention, and problem solving. These alcohol-related changes in the brain may be present even in babies whose appearance and growth are not affected. It is not known if there is any safe drinking level during pregnancy; nor is there any stage of pregnancy in which drinking—at any level—is known to be risk free. **If a woman is pregnant, or wants to become pregnant, she should not drink alcohol.** Even if she is pregnant and already has consumed alcohol, it is important to stop drinking for the rest of her pregnancy. Stopping can reduce the chances that her child might be harmed by alcohol.

Another risk of drinking is that a woman may at some point abuse alcohol or become alcoholic (alcohol dependent). Drinking four or more drinks on any given day OR drinking eight or more drinks in a typical week increases a woman's risk of developing alcohol abuse or dependence.

> The ability to drink a man—or anyone—under the table is not a plus: it is a red flag. Research has shown that drinkers who are able to handle a lot of alcohol all at once are at higher—not lower—risk of developing problems, such as dependence on alcohol.

Heavy Drinking

An estimated 5.3 million women in the United States drink in a way that threatens their health, safety, and general well-being. A strong case can be made that heavy drinking is more risky for women than men:

- *Heavy drinking increases a woman's risk of becoming a victim of violence and sexual assault.*

- *Drinking over the long term is more likely to damage a woman's health than a man's, even if the woman has been drinking less alcohol or for a shorter length of time than the man.*

The health effects of alcohol abuse and alcoholism are serious. Some specific health problems include:

- *Alcoholic liver disease:* Women are more likely than men to develop alcoholic hepatitis (liver inflammation) and to die from cirrhosis.

- *Brain disease:* Most alcoholics have some loss of mental function, reduced brain size, and changes in the function of brain cells. Research suggests that women are more vulnerable than men to alcohol-induced brain damage.

- *Cancer:* Many studies report that heavy drinking increases the risk of breast cancer. Alcohol also is linked to cancers of the digestive track and of the head and neck (the risk is especially high in smokers who also drink heavily).

- *Heart disease:* Chronic heavy drinking is a leading cause of cardiovascular disease. Among heavy drinkers, women are more susceptible to alcohol-related heart disease, even though women drink less alcohol over a lifetime than men.

Finally, many alcoholics smoke; smoking in itself can cause serious long-term health consequences.

Alcohol in Women's Lives:
Safe Drinking Over a Lifetime

The pressures to drink *more than what is safe*—and the consequences—change as the roles that mark a woman's life span change. Knowing the signs that drinking may be a problem instead of a pleasure can help women who choose to drink do so without harm to themselves or others.

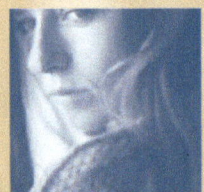

Adolescence

Despite the fact that drinking is illegal for anyone under the age of 21, the reality is that **many** adolescent girls drink. Research shows that about 37 percent of 9th grade girls—usually about 14 years old—report drinking in the past month. (This rate is slightly more than that for 9th grade boys.) Even more alarming is the fact that about 17 percent of these same young girls report having had five or more drinks on a single occasion during the previous month.

Consequences of Unsafe Drinking

- Drinking under age 21 is illegal in every State.

- Drunk driving is one of the leading causes of teen death.

- Drinking makes young women more vulnerable to sexual assault and unsafe and unplanned sex. On college campuses, assaults, unwanted sexual advances, and unplanned and unsafe sex are all more likely among students who drink heavily on occasion—for men, five drinks in a row, for women, four. In general, when a woman drinks to excess she is more likely to be a target of violence or sexual assault.

- Young people who begin drinking before age 15 have a 40-percent higher risk of developing alcohol abuse or alcoholism some time in their lives than those who wait until age 21 to begin drinking. This increased risk is the same for young girls as it is for boys.

Alcohol's Appeal for Teens. Among the reasons teens give most often for drinking are to have a good time, to experiment, and to relax or relieve tension. Peer pressure can encourage drinking. Teens who grow up with parents who support, watch over, and talk with them are less likely to drink than their peers.

Staying Away From Alcohol. Young women under age 21 should not drink alcohol. Among the most important things parents can do is to talk frankly with their daughters about not drinking alcohol.

Women in Young and Middle Adulthood

Young women in their twenties and early thirties are more likely to drink than older women. No one factor predicts whether a woman will have problems with alcohol, or at what age she is most at risk. However, there are some life experiences that seem to make it more likely that women will have drinking problems.

Heavy drinking and drinking problems among White women are most common in younger age groups. Among African American women, however, drinking problems are more common in middle age than youth. A woman's ethnic origins—and the extent to which she adopts the attitudes of mainstream vs. her native culture—influence how and when she will drink. Hispanic women who are more "mainstream" are more likely to drink and to drink heavily (that is, to drink at least once a week and to have five or more drinks at one time).

Research suggests that women who have trouble with their closest relationships tend to drink more than other women. Heavy drinking is more common among women who have never married, are living unmarried with a partner, or are divorced or separated. (The effect of divorce on a woman's later drinking may depend on whether she is already drinking heavily in her marriage.) A woman whose husband drinks heavily is more likely than other women to drink too much.

Many studies have found that women who suffered childhood sexual abuse are more likely to have drinking problems.

Depression is closely linked to heavy drinking in women, and women who drink at home alone are more likely than others to have later drinking problems.

Stress and Drinking

Stress is a common theme in women's lives. Research confirms that one of the reasons people drink is to help them cope with stress. However, it is not clear just how stress may lead to problem drinking. Heavy drinking by itself causes stress in a job and family. Many factors, including family history, shape how much a woman will use alcohol to cope with stress. A woman's past and usual drinking habits are important. Different people have different expectations about the effect of alcohol on stress. How a woman handles stress, and the support she has to manage it, also may affect whether she uses alcohol in response to stress.

- The number of female drivers involved in alcohol-related fatal traffic crashes is going up, even as the number of male drivers involved in such crashes has decreased. This trend may reflect the increasing number of women who drive themselves, even after drinking, as opposed to riding as a passenger.

- Long-term health problems from heavy drinking include liver, heart, and brain disease; suppression of the immune system; and cancer.

- Because women are more likely to become pregnant in their twenties and thirties, this age group faces the greatest risk of having babies with the growth and mental impairments of fetal alcohol syndrome, which is caused by drinking during pregnancy.

Older Women

As they grow older, fewer women drink. At the same time, research suggests that people born in recent decades are more likely to drink—throughout life—than people born in the early 1900s. Elderly patients are admitted to hospitals about as often for alcohol-related causes as for heart attacks.

Older women may be especially sensitive to the stigma of being alcoholic, and therefore hesitate to admit if they have a drinking problem.

Consequences of Unsafe Drinking

- Older women, more than any other group, use medications that can affect mood and thought, such as those for anxiety and depression. These "psychoactive" medications can interact with alcohol in harmful ways.

- Research suggests that women may be more likely to develop or to show alcohol problems later in life, compared with men.

Age and Alcohol. Aging seems to reduce the body's ability to adapt to alcohol. Older adults reach higher blood levels of alcohol even when drinking the same amount as younger people. This is because, with aging, the amount of water in the body is reduced and alcohol becomes more concentrated. But even at the same blood alcohol level, older adults may feel some of the effects of alcohol more strongly than younger people.

Alcohol problems among older people often are mistaken for other aging-related conditions. As a result, alcohol problems may be missed and untreated by health care providers, especially in older women.

Staying Well. Older women need to be aware that alcohol will "go to their head" more quickly than when they were younger. Also, caregivers need to know that alcohol may be the cause of problems assumed to result from age, such as depression, sleeping problems, eating poorly, heart failure, and frequent falls.

The National Institute on Alcohol Abuse and Alcoholism recommends that people ages 65 and older limit their consumption of alcohol to one drink per day.

An important point is that older people with alcohol problems respond to treatment as well as younger people. Those with shorter histories of problem drinking do better in treatment than those with long-term drinking problems.

Fewer women than men drink. However, among the heaviest drinkers, women equal or surpass men in the number of problems that result from their drinking. For example, female alcoholics have death rates 50 to 100 percent higher than those of male alcoholics, including deaths from suicides, alcohol-related accidents, heart disease and stroke, and liver cirrhosis.

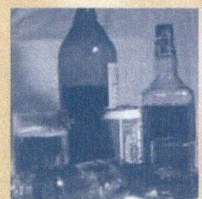

An Individual Decision

A woman's genetic makeup shapes how quickly she feels the effects of alcohol, how pleasant drinking is for her, and how drinking alcohol over the long term will affect her health, even the chances that she could have problems with alcohol. A family history of alcohol problems, a woman's risk of illnesses like heart disease and breast cancer, medications she is taking, and age are among the factors for each woman to weigh in deciding when, how much, and how often to drink.

What Are Alcohol Abuse and Alcoholism?

Alcohol abuse is a pattern of drinking that is harmful to the drinker or others. The following situations, occurring repeatedly in a 12-month period, would be indicators of alcohol abuse:

- Missing work or skipping child care responsibilities because of drinking

- Drinking in situations that are dangerous, such as before or while driving

- Being arrested for driving under the influence of alcohol or for hurting someone while drunk

- Continuing to drink even though there are ongoing alcohol-related tensions with friends and family.

Alcoholism or alcohol dependence is a disease. It is chronic, or life-long, and it can be both progressive and life threatening. Alcoholism is based in the brain. Alcohol's short-term effects on the brain are what cause someone to feel high, relaxed, or sleepy after drinking. In some people, alcohol's long-term effects can change the way the brain reacts to alcohol, so that the urge to drink can be as compelling as the hunger for food. Both a person's genetic makeup and his or her environment contribute to the risk for alcoholism. The following are some of the typical characteristics of alcoholism:

- *Craving:* a strong need, or compulsion, to drink

- *Loss of control:* the inability to stop drinking once a person has begun

- *Physical dependence:* withdrawal symptoms, such as nausea, sweating, shakiness, and anxiety, when alcohol use is stopped after a period of heavy drinking

- *Tolerance:* the need for increasing amounts of alcohol to get "high."

Know the Risks

Research suggests that a woman is more likely to drink excessively if she has any of the following:

- Parents and siblings (or other blood relatives) with alcohol problems

- A partner who drinks heavily

- The ability to "hold her liquor" more than others

- A history of depression

- A history of childhood physical or sexual abuse.

The presence of any of these factors is a good reason to be especially careful with drinking.

How Do You Know if You Have a Problem?

Answering the following four questions can help you find out if you or someone close to you has a drinking problem.

- Have you ever felt you should cut down on your drinking?

- Have people annoyed you by criticizing your drinking?

- Have you ever felt bad or guilty about your drinking?

- Have you ever had a drink first thing in the morning to steady your nerves or to get rid of a hangover?

One "yes" answer suggests a possible alcohol problem. If you responded "yes" to more than one question, it is very likely that you have a problem with alcohol. In either case, it is important that you see your health care provider right away to discuss your responses to these questions.

Even if you answered "no" to all of the above questions, if you are having drinking-related problems with your job, relationships, health, or with the law, you should still seek help.

Treatment for Alcohol Problems

Treatment for an alcohol problem depends on its severity. Women who have alcohol problems but who are not yet alcohol dependent may be able to stop or reduce their drinking with minimal help. Routine doctor visits are an ideal time to discuss alcohol use and its potential problems. Health care providers can help a woman take a good hard look at what effect alcohol is having on her life and can give advice on ways to stop drinking or to cut down.

RESEARCH DIRECTIONS

The National Institute on Alcohol Abuse and
Alcoholism (NIAAA), a component of the
National Institutes of Health (NIH), supports
about 90 percent of the Nation's research on
alcohol use and its effects. The goal of this
research is to better understand the causes and
consequences of alcohol abuse and addiction,
and to find new ways to prevent and treat
alcohol problems.

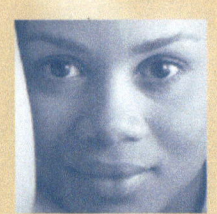

Finding out what makes some women drink too much is the first step to
preventing alcohol problems in women. Scientists are studying the role
of genetics and family environment in increasing or decreasing the risk
of alcohol problems. They also are studying other features of a woman's
life, such as the type of job she has; whether she combines family and work;
life changes like marriage, divorce, and the birth and departure of children;
infertility; relationship and sexual problems; and ethnic background.

Scientists want to know why women in general seem to develop long-
term health problems from drinking more quickly than men. Researchers
are examining issues like alcohol and breast cancer in women, and the
extent to which alcohol may lower the risk of heart disease, and possibly
osteoporosis, in some women.

Finally, research is helping determine how to identify women who may be
at risk for alcohol problems, and to ensure that treatment will be effective.

The Office of Research on Women's Health (ORWH) serves as the focal point for women's health research at NIH. ORWH works in a variety of ways to encourage and support researchers to find answers to questions about diseases and conditions that affect women and how to keep women healthy, and to establish a research agenda for the future. ORWH encourages women of all racial and ethnic backgrounds to participate in clinical studies to help increase knowledge of the health of women of all cultures, and to understand the health-related similarities and differences between women and men. The office also provides opportunities and support for the advancement of women in biomedical careers.

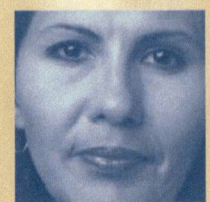

Alcoholics Anonymous (AA) World Services
Internet address: www.aa.org
Phone: 212–870–3400

Makes referrals to local AA groups and provides informational materials on the AA program. Many cities and towns also have a local AA office listed in the telephone book.

Al-Anon Family Group Headquarters
Internet address: www.al-anon.alateen.org
For locations of Al-Anon or Alateen meetings worldwide, call
888–4AL–ANON (888–425–2666), Monday through Friday,
8 a.m.–6 p.m. (EST)
For free informational materials, call 757–563–1600,
Monday through Friday, 8 a.m.–6 p.m.

Makes referrals to local Al-Anon groups, which are support groups for spouses and other significant adults in an alcoholic person's life. Also makes referrals to Alateen groups, which offer support to children of alcoholics.

National Association for Children of Alcoholics (NACoA)
Internet address: www.nacoa.net
E-mail: nacoa@nacoa.org
Phone: 888–554–COAS or 301–468–0985

Works on behalf of children of alcohol- and drug-dependent parents.

National Clearinghouse for Alcohol and Drug Information (NCADI)
Internet address: www.ncadi.samhsa.gov
Phone: 800–729–6686

Provides alcohol and drug abuse information produced by the Substance Abuse and Mental Health Services Administration, U.S. Department of Health and Human Services.

National Council on Alcoholism and Drug Dependence (NCADD)
Internet address: www.ncadd.org
Phone: 800–NCA–CALL (800–622–2255)

Provides telephone numbers of local NCADD affiliates (who can provide information on local treatment resources) and educational materials on alcoholism.

National Institute on Alcohol Abuse and Alcoholism (NIAAA)
5635 Fishers Lane, MSC 9304
Bethesda, Maryland 20892–9304
Internet address: www.niaaa.nih.gov
Phone: 301–443–3860

Offers a free 12-minute video, Alcohol: A Woman's Health Issue, *profiling women recovering from alcohol problems and describing the health consequences of heavy drinking in women. Other publications also are available from NIAAA and feature information on a wide variety of topics, including fetal alcohol syndrome, the dangers of mixing alcohol with medications, family history of alcoholism, and preventing underage drinking. See "Additional Reading," on page 20, for information on ordering NIAAA materials.*

Substance Abuse Treatment Facility Locator
Internet address: www.findtreatment.samhsa.gov
Phone: 800–662–HELP (800–662–4357)

Offers alcohol and drug information and treatment referral assistance. (This service is provided by the Substance Abuse and Mental Health Services Administration, U.S. Department of Health and Human Services.)

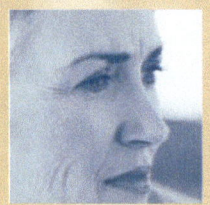

A Family History of Alcoholism: Are You at Risk?—offers easy-to-read information for anyone who is concerned about a family history of alcoholism. English version: NIH Publication Number 03–5340; Spanish version: NIH Publication Number 04–5340–S.

Drinking and Your Pregnancy—explains how drinking can hurt a developing baby, the problems that children born with fetal alcohol syndrome have, how to stop drinking, and where to go for help. English version: NIH Publication Number 96–4101; Spanish version: NIH Publication Number 97–4102.

Make a Difference: Talk to Your Child About Alcohol—offers guidance to parents and caregivers of young people ages 10 to 14 on preventing underage drinking. English version: NIH Publication Number 06–4314; Spanish version: NIH Publication Number 06–4314–S.

Tips for Cutting Down on Drinking—offers a checklist for reducing drinking, including setting goals and keeping track, tips for handling the urge to drink, and learning how to say "no" to alcohol. English and Spanish versions: excerpted from NIH Publication Number 07-3769.

To order, write to: National Institute on Alcohol Abuse and Alcoholism, Publications Distribution Center, P.O. Box 10686, Rockville, MD 20849–0686. The full text of all of the above publications is available on NIAAA's Web site (www.niaaa.nih.gov).

For more information on
alcohol abuse and alcoholism,
go to www.niaaa.nih.gov.
For more information on
women's health research, go
to http://orwh.od.nih.gov

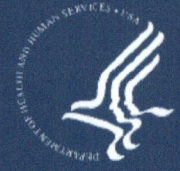
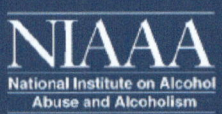

U.S. DEPARTMENT OF HEALTH AND HUMAN SERVICES
National Institutes of Health
National Institute on Alcohol Abuse and Alcoholism
NIH Publication No. 03 4956
Revised 2008

www.ingramcontent.com/pod-product-compliance
Lightning Source LLC
Chambersburg PA
CBHW061050290526
45796CB00002B/11